Doc Calloway works in a minor public school. Minor in terms of status but not in its teaching.

Gordon Calloway went to the school immediately after university, to be Head of Science, and has made biology his specialism. He claims that nothing gives greater pleasure than teaching science. This now includes girls as well as boys, of course, especially at sixth form level.

'Doc' is married and has children.

THE RESPIRATORY SYSTEM

Gordon Calloway, PhD

THE RESPIRATORY SYSTEM

EMMA
STERN
PUBLISHING

An Emma Stern Publication

A CIP catalogue record for this title is available from the British Library.

ISBN: 978-1-911224-12-9

Published in 2016

Emma Stern Publishing
107 Fleet Street
London
EC4A 2AB

www.emmastern.com
www.facebook.com/emmasternpublishing
Email: editorial@emmastern.com
Email: marketing@emmastern.com

Printed in Great Britain

This book, and companion volumes, has been set out in such a way that students and the general reader can learn quickly and easily.

In the case of students, the format is also eminently suitable for revision and for successfully tackling internal or external tests and examinations.

Useful for those studying:

* Biology;

* Human biology;

* Nursing;

* Community Health Care courses.

The respiratory system: anatomy

Look at this diagram, and keep referring to it as you read.

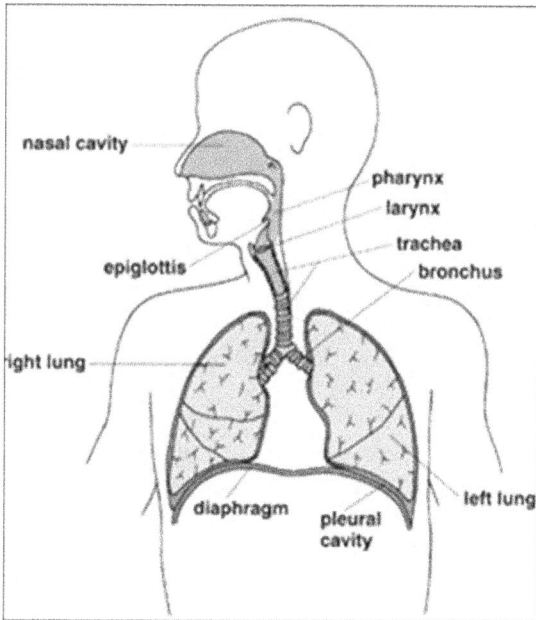

The Respiratory System has a large anatomy but the main organ is the lungs. The lungs are in the thorax (chest) protected by:

* the rib cage;

* the pleura

Nasal Cavity

As the air is breathed in through the nose, the air is warmed making it readier for inside our bodies.

As the air is breathed in through the nose, the air is warmed. The warmth is from blood vessels called capillaries, which are plentiful in the nose – as any boxer or playground scrapper will tell you!

To clean or filter the air there are:

A   *villi*

These are hair-like structures that line the respiratory tract from the nose down to the bronchioles.

B   *lymphatic tissues*

That combat bacteria and viruses, organised as nodes, of which the largest in the respiratory system are the adenoids and the tonsils.

Pharynx

The air continues to be warmed by the Pharynx.

The adenoids, protective lymph tissue, are found here.

So too are tonsils, situated further down the tract.

Larynx

Air passes through and on down to the Trachea

    The larynx is the voice box.

Trachea

When the air reaches the Trachea, it is protected behind the sternum (breast bone).

    The common name is wind pipe.

Bronchi

The trachea branches into two bronchi, each about the same length as the the trachea, and filtered air passes to the bronchioles.

Bronchioles

Each bronchus divides further into bronchioles and here air is passed through a branched system of passages inside the lungs.

Alveoli

These Alveoli are analogous to leaves on the branches of trees.

Each alveolus is surrounded by capillaries.

It is here that there is gaseous exchange, principally between oxygen and carbon dioxide.

There is also water vapour.

Gaseous exchange

The purpose of the lungs is to allow an exchange of gases.

The lungs contain about 300 million alveoli, representing a total surface area of 70-90 square metres, each wrapped in a fine mesh of capillaries.

The alveoli have single-celled epithelium. There is an extra-cellular matrix surrounded by capillaries.

There are 3 major alveolar cell types in the alveolar wall.

* cells that form the structure of an alveolar wall (pneumocytes).

* cells that secrete surfactant to lower the surface tension of water and allows the

membrane to separate thereby allowing gaseous exchange.

* cells that destroy foreign material, such as bacteria.

BUT........Alveoli have an innate tendency to collapse because of:

* their spherical shape,
* small size,
* surface tension due to water vapour.

Phospholipids help to equalize pressures and prevent collapse.

Phospholipids belong to the lipid family of fatty biological polymers.

A phospholipid is composed of two fatty acids, a glycerol unit, a phosphate group and a polar molecule.

Phospholipids are a major component of cell membranes. These membranes enclose the cytoplasm and other contents of a cell.

Phospholipids form a lipid bilayer.

This lipid bilayer is semi-permeable, allowing only certain molecules to diffuse across the membrane to enter or exit the cell.

What drives gaseous exchange?

Which gases are involved in the exchange?

Oxygen moves from the alveoli, which have a high oxygen concentration, to the blood, which has a lower oxygen concentration.

Why? Because oxygen is constantly being used and the concentrations must be equalised.

Conversely, carbon dioxide is produced by metabolism and has a higher concentration in the blood than in the air.

Oxygen in the lungs first diffuses through the alveolar wall and dissolves in the blood. The amount of oxygen dissolved in the fluid phase is governed by Henry's Law.

Oxygen dissolved in the blood diffuses into red blood cells and binds to haemoglobin, an iron compound.

The binding of oxygen to haemoglobin allows a greater amount of oxygen to be transported in the blood.

Although carbon dioxide and oxygen are the most important molecules exchanged, other gases are also transported between the alveoli and blood.

The amount of a gas that is exchanged depends on the water solubility of the gas and the affinity of the gas for haemoglobin.

Water vapour is also excreted through the lungs, due to humidification of inspired air by the lung tissues.

Henry's Law

Gases dissolve in liquids to form solutions. This dissolution is an equilibrium process for which an equilibrium constant can be written. For example, the equilibrium between oxygen gas and dissolved oxygen in water is $O_2(aq)$ <--> $O_2(g)$.

The equilibrium constant for this equilibrium is $K = p(O_2)/c(O_2)$.

The form of the equilibrium constant shows that the concentration of a solute gas in a solution is directly proportional to the partial pressure of that gas above the solution.

Henry's law is an accurate description of the behaviour of gases dissolving in liquids when concentrations and partial pressures are reasonably low. As concentrations and partial pressures increase, deviations from Henry's law become noticeable. This behaviour is very similar to the behaviour of gases, which are found to deviate from the norm as pressures increase and temperatures decrease. For this reason, solutions which are found to obey Henry's law are sometimes called ideal dilute solutions.

What is a pneumothorax?

A pneumothorax is a collapsed lung.

It can be caused by:

a fractured rib;

trauma from knife, bullet, etc.

Risk factors are cigarette smoking and drug abuse.

Spontaneous pneumothorax

This refers to a condition in which the lung collapses with no apparent injury or trauma.

The alveoli collapse and leak air into the pleural spaces, making breathing difficult.

Disease-related pneumothorax can occur due to abnormalities in the lung tissue.

Examples are:

* asthma

* pulmonary disease - congestion

* emphysema - over-inflation of the alveoli

* chronic bronchitis

* diseases such as AIDS.

Atmospheric & pulmonary air

Atmospheric (external) air contains a high percentage of oxygen and nitrogen.

Alveolar gas contains a lower percentage of oxygen and a higher percentage of carbon dioxide.

The differences in composition are due to the fact that gaseous exchange is taking place within the alveoli in the lungs.

Oxygen diffuses from the alveoli into the pulmonary artery and carbon dioxide diffuses back into the alveoli from the pulmonary artery due to the concentration gradients. This is the main reason why external air and alveolar gas have different compositions.

Another reason is the fact that alveolar gas contains a mixture of both atmospheric air which has been inhaled and 'old' air which stays in the respiratory tract and is not exhaled after each breath therefore giving it a different composition.

Alveolar gas has more moisture, because it is warmed and moistened in its passage to the lungs.

Vocabulary

Check the meanings of the following terms, all mentioned in the book.

Write down a short definition of each one.

pleura

epithelium

matrix

capillaries

polymers

polar molecule

diffusion

dissolution

constant

www.ingramcontent.com/pod-product-compliance
Lightning Source LLC
Chambersburg PA
CBHW020757220326
41520CB00051B/585